THE SCR
HANDI

G000096144

A Practitioner's Guide

by
John Fry
General Practitioner

Pauline Jeffree
Practice Nurse

and
Kenneth Scott
*General Practitioner,
Beckenham, Kent*

KLUWER ACADEMIC PUBLISHERS
DORDRECHT / BOSTON / LONDON

Distributors

---

for the United States and Canada: Kluwer Academic Publishers, PO Box 358, Accord Station, Hingham, MA 02018-0358, USA
for all other countries: Kluwer Academic Publishers Group, Distribution Center, PO Box 322, 3300 AH Dordrecht, The Netherlands

British Library Cataloguing in Publication Data

Fry, John, *1922–*
    The screening handbook.
    1. Man. Chronic diseases. Diagnosis. Screening
    I. Title   II. Jeffree, Pauline   III. Scott, Kenneth
    616.07'5

    ISBN 0-7923-8926-3

Published in the United Kingdom by Kluwer Academic Publishers, PO Box 55, Lancaster, UK.

Kluwer Academic Publishers BV incorporates the publishing programmes of D. Reidel, Martinus Nijhoff, Dr W. Junk and MTP Press.

Printed in Great Britain by Butler and Tanner Ltd., Frome and London.

CONTENTS

Chapter 1

BASICS

AIMS OF CARE

The basic aims of medical care are as old as time itself, namely:

– to *cure* sometimes
– to *relieve* often
– to *comfort* always

Now that many diseases are curable and controllable, the emphasis of care is shifting towards:

– *prevention* of *disease*
– *promotion* of *health*

These objectives are now enshrined in the 'new general practice' and are included in the White Paper and New Contract for general practice of 1989.

GENERAL PRACTICE: KEY ROLES

The general practitioner and the whole practice team have important roles and opportunities in these policies of health promotion and disease prevention for reasons that follow:

– the general practitioner is known and respected by patients as a personal and family doctor

1

– the practice team is available and accessible to patients daily

– the GP sees over two-thirds of his patients at least once a year and on average the consultation rate is 3–4 consultations per person per year

– therefore, the GP sees most of his patients annually and many on a number of occasions and over a period of 5 years over 90% of patients will be seen

– with a relatively stable population, the general practitioner and team are able to provide long term and continuing care.

Therefore, for all these reasons the general practice has opportunities to act, but in acting there must be achievable short term and long term objectives and feasible plans.

PRINCIPLES

There are roles for patients as well as the team in prevention of disease, and promotion of health, and both have to collaborate and cooperate.

– *patients* have responsibilities in following basic health habits such as avoidance of smoking and excess alcohol, and taking a reasonable diet and undertaking regular exercise. They should be prepared to manage minor illness themselves and to cooperate and comply with doctors in long term care of chronic illness and to consult early for appropriate symptoms and signs.

– to achieve such goals, the public has to be suitably informed and educated.

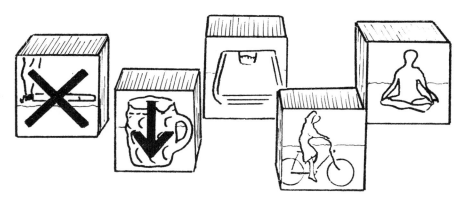

Building towards a healthy life

– for the *practice team*, educating and informing patients on prevention of disease and health maintenance should be carried out whenever and wherever possible in order to change bad habits and encourage self-help and self-reliance.

– a priority of good medical practice has to be an early and accurate clinical diagnosis in order to prevent progression of disease processes through effective treatment.

WHAT IS 'SCREENING'?

Screening is not something new and technical. Unknowingly it has always been an integral part of good general practice for, as well as endeavouring to detect and diagnose early and to sort out what requires specific treatment and what can be left to get better naturally, the general practitioner will enquire on personal habits and health risks and encourage a healthy life

3

style, and as a family doctor he will be aware of particular possible familial tendencies such as early death from vascular diseases, diabetes and even personality problems.

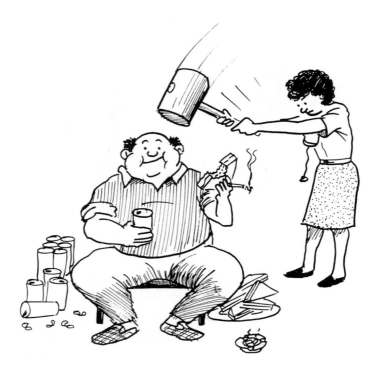

Aversion therapy

Recently an extension of these principles has been the setting up of screening clinics to pick up preventable disorders at their pre-symptomatic stages and to try and correct unhealthy habits before they do harm.

POLICIES IN PRACTICE

These ideals need to be incorporated into the busy life of everyday general practice but this requires sensitive and sensible understanding and planning.

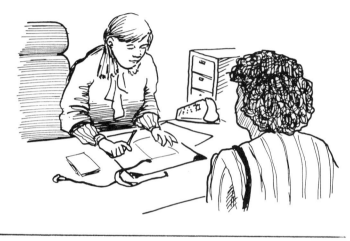

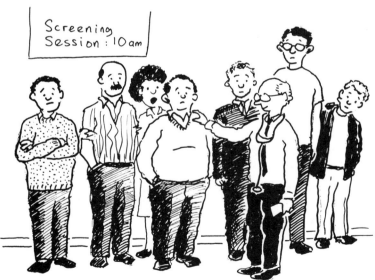

"You'll have to excuse Dr Jones — he used to be a police surgeon"

– *every routine consultation* offers opportunities on enquiry, advice and counselling, on health promotion in addition to the presenting clinical problems.

– as noted *special specific 'screening' exercises* can be organised to detect those patients at risk and plan their appropriate personal management but these clinics require careful planning and action to be effective.

REALITIES

All these philosophies are fine, but it has to be remembered that:

– the GP is a very busy person!

– he has little spare time to take on new work unless it is demonstrated that it is really useful.

– he has to be convinced that on balance prevention and healthy promotion through personal health education and through screening exercises should have a high priority in competition with so many other tasks.

– achievement of goals can only be reached through good cooperation between patients and the whole practice team.

Success of any screening exercise depends on careful attention to details.

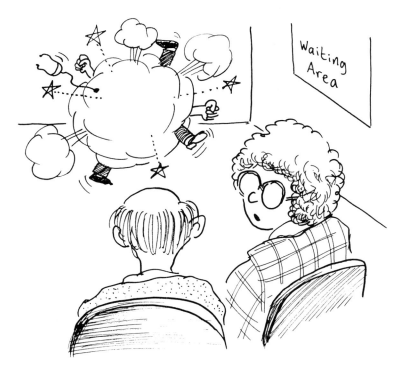

*"I think I'll come back after they've been on
their team building course"*

PRELIMINARY STEPS

– Screening is a composite exercise involving the whole
  practice – doctors, staff and patients – and there should be
  general agreement on aims and objectives which should be
  incorporated into practice policies.

– The basic issues on which agreement is necessary are:

WHO does WHAT, WHY, WHERE, WHEN and HOW?

SETTING UP

– To repeat, 'screening' should be *opportunistic* during every suitable consultation, but for it to be successful, there should be guidelines to remind those involved on what should be checked and recorded, such as questions on smoking and drinking habits, weight and blood pressure measurements at least once every 5 years.

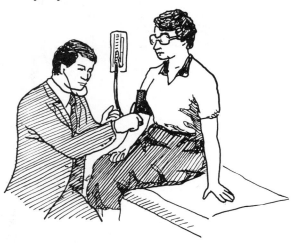

– *formal screening* involves setting up programmes with attention to plans and protocols.

WHO should be involved?

– *doctors* should be involved in planning and in carrying out, or supervising, clinical procedures, measurements and analysis of results.

– *practice nurses, health visitors and district nurses* will be involved in planning, face-to-face procedures and recording.

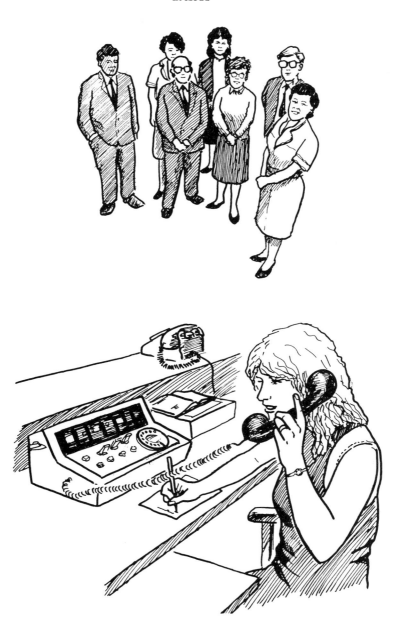

The Receptionist – an important part of the team

- *practice managers and receptionists* will be concerned with the general organisation.

- *patients* are what screening is all about and they have to be involved at all stages.

WHAT methods?

Planning should include attention to:

- *screening records* – decisions have to be made on whether they should be part of the normal NHS record or specially prepared and filed separately.

- *computers* – are being used increasingly and their potential must be realised and exploited (see pages 121–2).

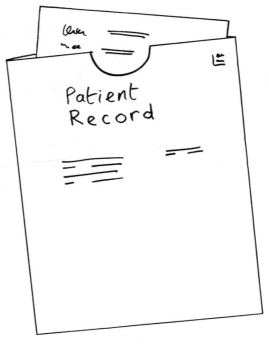

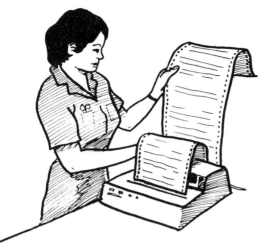

- *other tools and equipment* – have to be relatively easy to use, reliable and validated to yield accurate information.

- *costs* must be realistic and it is important to estimate what is likely to be involved and the costs and whether they can be met through approved NHS items of service such as cervical cytology, updating of immunisations against tetanus (see also Chapter 5).

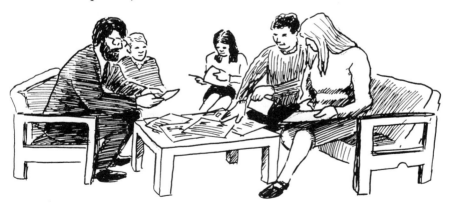

Preparing the Practice Information Leaflet

– *communication within the practice* – is important, including exchange information, and arrangements for publicity, invitations to patients and arrangements for the clinics, and also to report regularly on success and on problems encountered.

FOLLOW-ON

The exercise does not end with the 'screening' exercise, good follow-up is essential.

– *Defaulters and non-attenders* must be chased up.

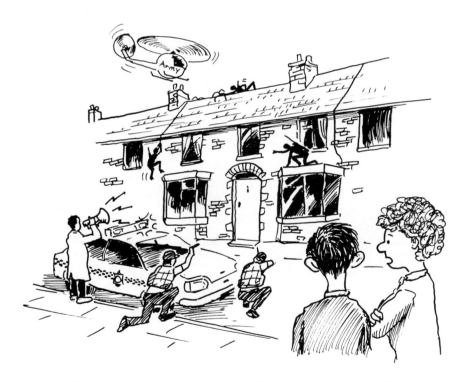

"I did warn him not to miss Dr Fry's screening clinic"

– *Follow-up* should include checks on health state, compliance in treatment and self-help in following advice on changing risk habits, such as smoking and drinking. Space for such follow-up assessments must be included on the records.

– *Audit and self-checks* must be carried out to try and measure improvements.

– *Cost-benefits* should also be assessed (where possible) to ensure that there has been 'value' for the money, time and efforts expended.

Chapter 2

SPECIFICS

To recap, the *aims* of screening must be part of our routine consultation process of good general practice, namely, to detect and diagnose early and institute appropriate care and at the same consultation be alert to possible personal health risks and to recommend lifestyle changes, if indicated. These same aims apply to the more formal screening process.

UNDERLYING PRINCIPLES

If a practice is to introduce formal screening then certain rules and principles should be followed and applied:

– all the practice team and staff have to agree that screening is worthwhile and beneficial, and commit themselves and be prepared to undertake allotted roles and tasks.

– screening programmes have to be selected and identified based on the interests of the practice and general policies defined and followed – ideally these should be produced by a small group and then discussed and approved at a practice meeting.

– those to be involved must understand and accept their roles.

– the resources required have to be worked out and costed and there has to be agreement to meet the costs (see pages 103–8).

- the patients (or client group) to be targeted must be defined and plans made to check their names and addresses.

- practice protocols for the screening programme have to be agreed, written out and followed, but with flexibility for changes.

- one or two 'pilot trials' should be carried out before the project starts.

- there should be measurable benefits for patients.

WHO TO SCREEN?

'Screening' can be used for a wide range of conditions and groups but in practice there are a few that will provide best value for effort. It is better in practice to target on patient (client) groups than on specific disorders such as high blood pressure or diabetes, because these should be picked up in the screening process.

Thus those recommended are:

- Ante-Natal Clinic

- Child Surveillance Clinic

- Well-Woman Clinic

- Well-Man Clinic

- Elderly (over 75 years)

- New Registrants

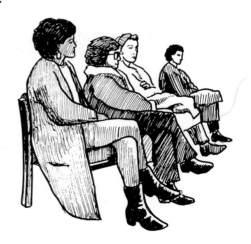

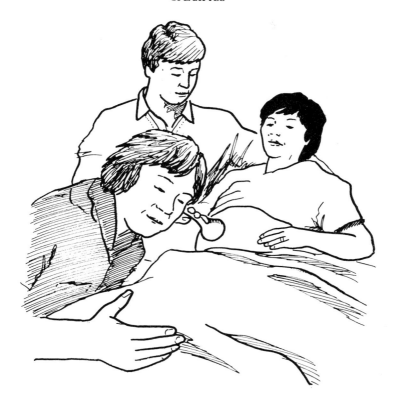

It is evident from this list that the top two, ante-natal and child surveillance, have been 'part of good practice for a long time'. Well-person clinics are more recent but probably appreciated by patients and value-for-effort; screening of elderly and new registrants are proposed in the new contract, their value-for-effort is uncertain but they have to be considered (see also pages 54–63).

General practice is well placed to provide mothercraft classes for their patients which can be organised by the practice and supported by the attached health visitor.

HOW TO IDENTIFY

Those to be screened here have to be identified and encouraged to attend. The identification can be achieved in various ways:

− from a practice *Age-Sex Register* if the targets are persons in certain age groups, i.e. over 75s or males 30–60 or teenagers. Naturally, the age-sex registers have to be up-to-date and accurate for current addresses.

− computer print-outs from the Family Practitioners Committee. This can be easily done for age and sex but fees now are levied for this service.

− from the practice computer − if one is available (see page 10).

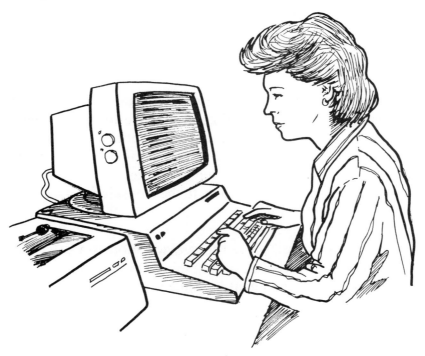

– from a practice disease-index – this provides unlimited opportunities for an assessment and follow-up of patients diagnosed or indexed by certain diseases who can be called up.

– record markers can be used short term to pick out those sought to be screened.

– opportunistically, patients can be invited as a result of consultations, from recalls for cervical cytology and at attendances for other reasons such as mothers seen for child surveillance or attending the surgery for other reasons.

FOR EACH GROUP

Whatever the group to be screened certain steps should be followed and checked.

Basic questions

– what is being screened for? There should be clear aims for the exercise at the start so that an evaluation can be made.

– who is to be screened? There has to be a definite target group that can be approached and invited.

– how to do it? The methods used should be relatively simple, reliable, comparable and possible of validation, and those using them should be trained and tested beforehand.

– how to monitor, achieve and evaluate? This has to be a part of each screening exercise (see Chapter 6).

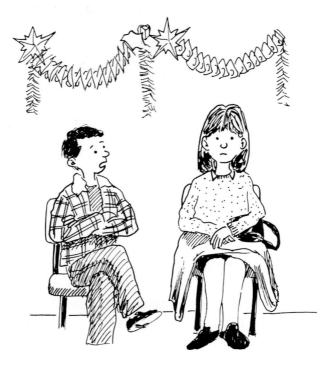

*"Actually, it does pay to come to all of her screening clinics
– I've just been invited to the Christmas party"*

Check list of details

Now that it is agreed that the screening exercise should go ahead there are important check points to note:

– someone has to be in overall charge to direct, plan and execute.

– timing has to be right for patients as well as staff, and sessions must not be too frequent or too distant.

- those identified have to be informed and appointments confirmed.

- those taking part must know what is expected and have tried and tested the procedures.

- facilities have to be available and equipment in place.

- do not be over-ambitious and be prepared for hiccups and frustrations.

DEFAULTERS

The aim of all screening programmes must be to achieve 100% attendance and experience shows this is virtually unachievable. A compromise has to be accepted and the practice must recognise this and aim at realistic targets.

Health screening is a new concept in the development of primary care and our patients have to become adjusted to this development. Until this has been achieved it must be recognised that failure to respond to invitations to attend screening programmes could be met with some degree of indifference. The practice needs to adopt a planned programme for those patients who fail to attend.

It is recommended that:

- no more than a second invitation be extended to defaulters.
- patients who fail to respond to the original invitation may respond to a second invitation if this is by personal contact.
- defaulters can be included in the screening programme oportunistically should this be appropriate.

SCREENING CARD

It is essential to include a screening card in the patient's medical record envelope, which will give the detailed results of the screening undertaken and also indicate failure to attend. The value of this system will include opportunistic screening to be undertaken when patients attend the surgery routinely in identifying recall.

Defaulters can be readily identified by the inclusion within the medical record of a pre-determined coloured marker which can be removed when the programme has been completed.

A system needs to be devised which allows for immediate identification of all patients who have attended screening programmes.

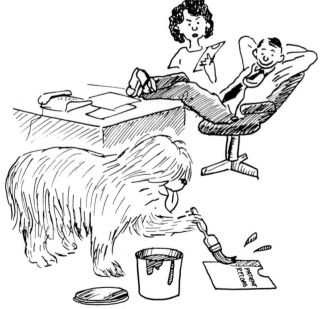

"You always have to be different –
Dr Jones does it with a felt-tip pen"

The use of a computer is the simplest method to record these data. A manual system, however, can be achieved by marking the outside of the patient's medical record envelope.

PROMOTION

A key factor is promotion through good relations and communication with patients. The exercise cannot succeed unless atients know that it is available and what are its aims.

In-practice 'advertising' has to be carried out extensively and enthusiastically. There are various opportunities:

- Surgery notice board
- Practice newsletter
- Specific invitations to targeted patients
- Personal contacts during consultations and at other opportunities
- Practice Interest Group
- Practice leaflet
- Practice staff and professional staff attached to the practice

HEALTH PROMOTION CLINICS

Thus there are three types of screening activities:

- *opportunitistic screening* as part of a consultation involving accurate early diagnosis and inquiry on possible lifestyle health risks.

- screening of *defined patient groups* such as ante-natals, child surveillance, well-person, elderly and new registrants.

- screening and support of *specific conditions* such as diabetes, high blood pressure and cardiovascular disorders, smokers (and anti-smoking clinics), alcoholics (and alcohol control), overweight and the stressed.

Here we describe our arrangements for some of the patient-group clinics, but the principles apply to others also.

We shall not deal with ante-natal and child surveillance clinics because they have been a part of general practice for many years, but we must make the point that they are complementary. Child care starts in the ante-natal period when receptive expectant mothers, especially primiparae, can receive advice and grounding from midwives and health visitors as well as general practitioners.

CHILD DEVELOPMENT AND SURVEILLANCE

Primary care services since 1974 are provided by the community health staff of the district health authority and by general practitioners, who have received specific training for this, and their team.

Child health and development

General practitioner or clinical medical officers, health visitor, practice nurse.

Call and recall

Many district health authorities are using a national child health computer system which consists of the following modules:

- a child register with neonatal data
- immunisation schedule
- pre-school health
- school health

The contents and programmes for screening 0–5 year old children vary.

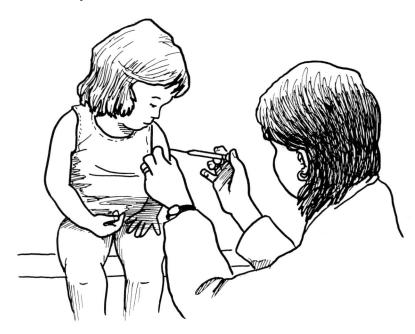

The following is a schedule recommended in the Court Report:

Age	Objectives
6–8 weeks	– assess mother and baby bonding – discuss feeding problems and check feeding – discuss immunisation programme – exclude congenital abnormalities such as dislocation of the hips – examine to make sure there is normal physical-neuro development – make sure the baby is registered with the practice
8–9 months	– carry out distraction hearing tests – determine whether the child can sit without support – assess manipulation skills – assess vision and test for squint
18 months	– ensure walking well – assess fine motor skills
2–3 years	– assess letter matching – vision testing – carry out word discrimination hearing test – assess speech and language – assess fine motor and performance skills

The child's physical development should be regularly plotted on a centile display chart.

Basic equipment for child health clinic

– standard centile chart to plot weight and head circumference and therefore growth for male and female

- baby scales
- baby measuring tape (paedometer), wall charts
- torch
- ophthalmoscope
- auroscope
- stethoscope
- red brick/ball
- child's table and chair to sit at
- Stycar vision and hearing box

WELL-MAN CLINICS

The objectives are to invite men in defined age groups to attend for interview and examination in order to assess their state of health and pick up any health risks in their lifestyles and seek to correct them.

Introduction

A well-man clinic can be undertaken (1) in either an entirely opportunistic way similar to the Oxford Heart Disease Prevention Project or (2) by an organised call programme for men in defined age groups.

- Male patients attending routine surgeries for consultation are invited to attend the well-man screening clinic operating concurrently at the surgery.

- Men within the identified age range agreed by the practice will be asked to see the practice nurse who is facilitating this clinic and the same procedure will be adopted as for that identified for the planned well-man clinic.

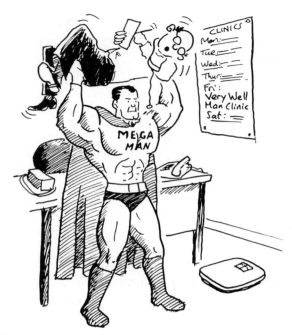

"Everything seems to be in order. I'll see you in 15 years."

The steps mentioned (pages 15–16) should be followed and a check list prepared and adhered to.

- Identify age range to be screened
- Whom to screen?
- Numbers to be called
- How many sessions required and how often?
- How many per session and how long?
- Organisation of invitations and reception
- Staff involved, roles and training
- What to do?
- How to evaluate?

About 15–20 minutes per patient is about right, but there should be a smooth flow with the practice team knowing their roles and tasks.

A *patient questionnaire* may be used (see page 47) and this can be sent out with an invitation and appointment for completion at home and delivery on attendance. Some repetition is inevitable, but replies can serve as double checks.

Allocation of tasks will vary from practice to practice. Our procedure is that a doctor is present on site at the time of each session and that the work is carried out by the practice nursing team.

1. *General health* including present state, past illnesses and any current medication.

2. *Family history* – near relatives, with particular note of cardiovascular diseases and early deaths.

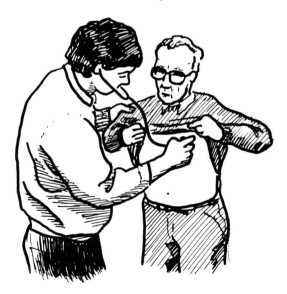

3. *Personal habits*
   - amount of regular exercise
   - smoking extent and duration (present and past)
   - alcohol – units per week
   - diet – amounts of salinated fats and fibre intake

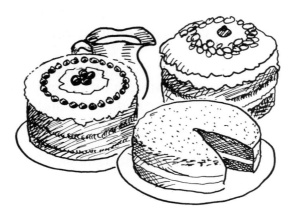

Nice – but naughty

4. *Personal data*
   - height
   - weight
   - blood pressure
   - urinalysis
   - peakflow measurement
   - blood cholesterol and triglycerides (but agreement necessary on levels at which various management options to be followed, and also make prior arrangements with local laboratory)

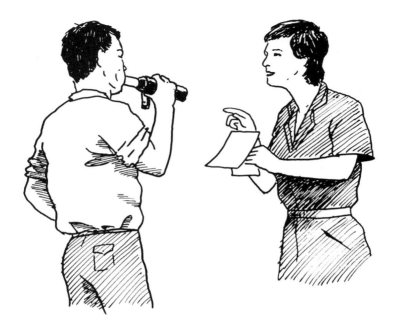

5. *Others*
   - immunisation state, particularly tetanus and polio
   - stress levels can be noted during consultation and also measured using psychiatric questionnaires
   - teach testicular self-examination

At the end of the screening a *heart chart* (overleaf) can be completed by the patient to give him indication of his at-risk state. This will also allow discussion at a follow-up consultation for those at risk.

Note

Updating patient's polio and tetanus status attract item of service fees at the present time.

HEALTH CHART TO BE COMPLETED BY PATIENT

Factor	0	1
Family history of high blood pressure or heart disease	None known	Possible but unsure
Diastolic blood pressure	Normal	85–90
Smoking	Non-smoker	Less than 5 a day
Fat in diet	No fried food Always use low fat foods	Fried food once a week, low fat foods most days
Weight	Normal	3.2–6.4 kg overweight
Alcohol (units/week where 1 unit = a half pint of beer/lager, one measure of spirit or glass of wine)	Men: 0–2 Women: 0–1	2–4 1–2
Stress	No more than usual	Occasional stress at home or work
Exercise	Three times or more a week	Twice a week

2	3	4
Extended family e.g. cousins	Immediate family – one relative	Immediate family – two or more relatives
91–95	96–100	Over 100
5–9	10–19	More than 20
Fried food twice a week, low fat food once a week	Fried food most days, low fat food occasionally	Fried food every day, never use low fat foods
6.4–9.5 kg overweight	9.5–12.7 kg overweight	12.7 kg or more overweight
4–6 2–3	6–8 3–4	2–8 or more 2–4 or more
Occasional stress at home and work	Considerable at home or work	Showing symptoms/on medication for stress
Once a week	Once every 2–4 weeks	Less than once a week

A QUICK INTERPRETATION OF THE SCORE FROM THE 'HEART CHART'

Score

21–40   ◯   *Danger:* Your lifestyle needs a major overhaul

11–20   ◯   *Caution:* There are several blackspots requiring servicing

0–10   ◯   *Proceed with care:* There may be hazards ahead

Name: _____

Your score is: _____

Areas to change: _____

_____

_____

Follow-up

It is recommended that the following procedures are undertaken as a result of well-man screening programmes.

– Patients should be reviewed on a 3-yearly basis.

– All patients considered to be at risk should be referred to the doctor and investigated and treated.

– Referral to specific clinics where changes in lifestyle have been recommended as part of promoting better health.

PRE-CONCEPTUAL CARE OR PRE-PREGNANCY HEALTH

It is recognised that the health of both parents at the time of conception is as important as the health of the expectant mother during pregnancy. Preparation for parenthood begins, therefore, before the baby is conceived.

There are some environmental factors, however, which whilst affecting an individual cannot be changed, such as pollution.

Perinatal mortality and morbidity rates have reduced, but these rates can still be improved. It is anticipated that pre-conceptual care will help in their reduction.

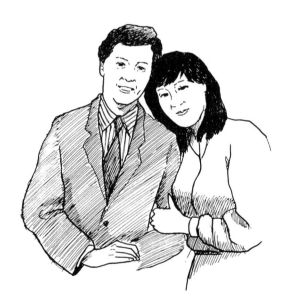

There are a number of factors which are known to affect the outcome of pregnancy:

- maternal age
- parity
- socio-economic status of the father of the baby
- maternal health

Pre-conceptual care is a means, whether such care is given on an ad hoc basis say at a family planning clinic or at pre-conceptual care clinics, of identifying problems, and referring where appropriate. The practice nurse in this situation is a health educator, a resource person and also uses her/his skills to identify problems.

Medical aspects of pre-conceptual care:

- blood test for Rubella status
- blood pressure
- weight
- height
- urine analysis
- blood profile
- cervical smear

Details of the health of both partners:

- general health
- lifestyle
- contraception
- eating habits

The above information provides a baseline from which to assess changes during pregnancy.

WELL-WOMAN CLINIC

The practice needs to agree that it wishes to run a well- woman clinic, that there are the resources for such a clinic and the facilities available to undertake the clinic.

It should also be agreed who will be responsible for the clinic and who will operate the clinic.

It is an ideal role for the practice nurse who could be delegated this task. It is essential that the practice nurse has had the appropriate training and has been assessed and authorised following practice protocols and treatment room policies, and if the nurse accepts the delegated task as part of her extended role, has a certificate of competence, duly signed and dated stating that the nurse is competent to carry out the procedure in question.

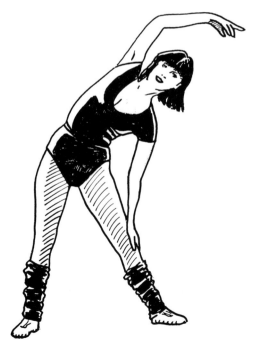

The United Kingdom Central Council for Nursing Midwifery and Health Visiting Document Code of Professional Conduct, 2nd Edition, November 1984, states:

"4. Acknowledge any limitations of competence and refuse in such cases to accept delegated functions without first having received instruction in regard to those functions and having been assessed as competent."

The overall responsibility for the clinic should be that of an identified partner in the practice who will be available on site at the time of the clinic should the nurse wish to refer for medical advice.

The objectives of a well-woman clinic are to invite women to attend for interview and examination in order to:

- assess their state of health
- identify health risks in their lifestyle
- examine the breasts and teach self examination of the breasts
- identify uterine/hormone function
- undertake a pelvic examination, inspect the cervix and take a cervical smear

Equipment

Special equipment required for well-woman clinics is identified in Chapter 4, Resources.

Unlike a well-man clinic it is inappropriate to undertake a well-woman's screening opportunistically as women need to be prepared for the examination that is included in the interview,

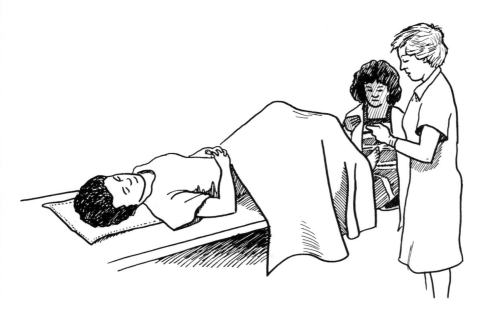

and because of the length of time that is required to be allocated to each examination (usually 20 minutes).

However, clinics can be organised on a self-referral basis.

Operation of the clinic

The target group should be identified by the use of computer or age sex register and invited to attend the clinic using the standard technique, see pages 18–19.

A detailed record needs to be kept of the outcome of each client who attends for the practice audit and as part of evaluation.

Procedure for establishing a well-woman clinic

The women invited to attend a well-woman clinic should be informed in advance of the procedures to be undertaken at the clinic.

Patients attending a well-woman clinic will be asked to complete a health questionnaire (see page 47) which will include details of lifestyle and uterine function. This questionnaire can be sent to the client prior to attending the clinic, with the explanatory leaflet.

At the clinic the practice nurse checks the completed questionnaire and interviews the patient. The patient should be put at her ease by the nurse explaining the procedure and discussing the health questionnaire.

Clinic organisation

The practice must agree the organisation of the clinic, who is to run the clinic and ensure that appropriate resources are made available.

This means:

– when it is to occur
– who is to run the clinic
– clerical and administrative support
– who is to pull the records of the clients attending
– where the clinic is to be held
– who is to invite the patient, and the form of the invitation
– who is to complete the forms

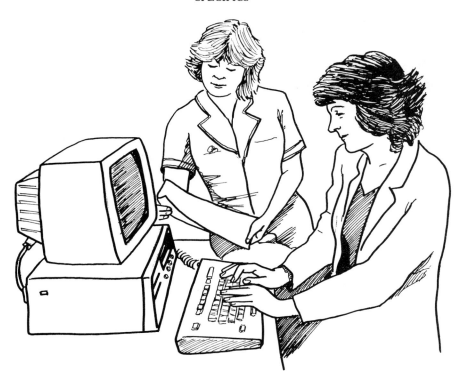

The clinic should be run by the practice nurse with the support of a partner in the practice, and an identified member of the clerical staff should be responsible for pulling the records for the client group identified by the practice.

The practice nurse should be responsible for screening the records of the patients included in the client group in order to eliminate those patients for whom it would be inappropriate for them to be invited, e.g. the severely disabled.

The clerical staff will complete any Path. and/or FPC claim forms.

The form of invitation should be designed and agreed by the practice team and the clerical staff should be responsible for extending the invitation to the identified patients offering them suitable appointments.

The location of the clinic should be agreed by the practice team and the practice nurse should be responsible for ensuring equipment is available at the time of the clinic.

Invitation to a well-woman lifestyle clinic

Dear Mrs ...

The practice has introduced a well-woman/lifestyle programme as part of the primary care service to the patients of the practice.

You are invited to attend the surgery to take part in this programme and I am enclosing an explanatory leaflet and a questionnaire which I would like you to complete prior to your appointment.

Will you please attend   on:
                        at:

Should this be inconvenient, please telephone the surgery to make an alternative appointment.

Yours sincerely,

Practice Nurse

Leaflet

Surgery Address

Dr.
Dr.
Dr.
Dr.

Practice Nurse
Practice Nurse
Practice Nurse

Well-Woman/Lifestyle Screening Programme

The purpose of this programme is to:

- Assess your current state of health
- Discuss your lifestyle

Your practice have established health care screening programmes which offers you the opportunity to discuss aspects of your health and lifestyle. Sister . . . . , who is as you know the practice nurse, will be undertaking the examination which will include height, weight, blood pressure, urine test, breast examination and cervical smear.

At the clinic you will have the opportunity to discuss with Sister any health care problem you may have. Should you be having a period at the time of your appointment please arrange to change your appointment for a more convenient time.

Please bring an early morning specimen of urine to your consultation.

Please allow at least 15–20 minutes for completion of the examination.

WELL-WOMAN HEALTH QUESTIONNAIRE

Please answer the following questions before you see the nurse.

1.	Do you consider you are in good health?		YES/NO
2.	Is there a family history of:	Heart disease	YES/NO
		Diabetes	YES/NO

3. Do you smoke? YES/NO
   If *YES* how many do you smoke a day? ......
   Have you tried to stop? YES/NO
   Do you wish to stop? YES/NO

4. Do you drink alcohol? YES/NO
   If *YES* how many units do you drink a day?......
   (half pint of lager or single spirit measure = 1 unit)

5. Do you self-examine your breasts regularly? YES/NO

6. Menstrual history
   - Do you have any period problems? YES/NO
   - Age of starting periods ....
   - Number of days of bleeding ....
   - Period interval (1st to last day) ....
   - Any change in cycle ....
   - Date of last period (for appropriate
     appointment) ....

7. Are you happy with your present method of
   contraception? YES/NO

8. Have you ever had a cervical smear? YES/NO

9. Have you had a recent: Tetanus booster? YES/NO
   Polio booster? YES/NO

Thank you for completing this questionnaire. Please give it to nurse at your consultation.

Case history

The patient aged 42 years self-referred to well-woman clinic.

The appropriate questionnaire was administered, completed and evaluated by the nurse and this indicated normal lifestyle, regular periods and no symptoms or apparent problems.

Height:	1.65 m
Weight	54 kg
Blood pressure:	120/75
Urine:	Nothing abnormal detected
Breasts:	Nil to find at time of examination. Self-examination of breasts taught
Pelvic examination:	Uterus appeared to be enlarged, inspection of the cervix showed a small fleshy lump extruding from the cervix. Cervical smear taken.

Patient referred to general practitioner who confirmed:

- the patient to have an enlarged uterus due to fibroids
- the presence of a cervical polyp

Clinical findings were explained to the patient and the appropriate referral was made to Gynaecology out-patients. Patient subsequently admitted where she had an examination under general anaesthetic, dilatation and curettage and removal of the cervical polyp.

Diagnostic curettage revealed no abnormality. The consultant opinion was not to undertake surgical intervention with regard to the fibroids as the patient was asymptomatic, and suggested an annual review.

Cervical smear reported inflammatory cells and it was requested that it be repeated in one year.

NEW ENTRANTS TO THE PRACTICE

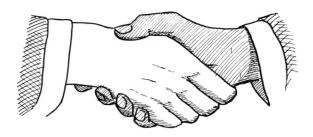

The New Contract proposes a *registration fee* for all new registrations (except the newly born) which will be paid to GPs who carry out certain specified procedures in respect of patients joining their lists for the first time.

This task is best undertaken by the practice nurse. Appointments should be offered to the patients when they join the list.

The most appropriate time to invite new patients to come for assessment is:

- In the evening, after 6 pm, for those people who work
- In the early morning, say 11 am, for women with young families, and the elderly
- Weekend appointments

The new entrants' interview with the practice nurse offers the ideal opportunity for patients to be welcomed into the practice prior to the nurse undertaking the basic screening programme.

The aim of this examination is:

- to identify the medical and social background of the patient
- to familiarise the patient with the activities and facilities within the practice:

- identifying the practice team
- appointments procedures
- specialist clinics
- repeat prescription protocol

The patient should complete a questionnaire and it should be reviewed by the practice nurse at interview.

We have used *new patient questionnaires* for some time.

NEW PATIENT QUESTIONNAIRE

This set of questions has been designed to help the practice health care team get to know you and any medical problems you may have.

The information will be treated confidentially. Should you wish not to answer any questions, please leave them blank.

It will be appreciated if you will kindly complete and return the questionnaire before you attend for your health screening check by our practice nurse.

Mr/Mrs/Miss/Ms   *Date of birth:*

Address: *Telephone No:*

Origin: (for haemoglobinopathies)

Occupation:

Childhood illnesses   Measles
                                          Age:

Asthma   Mumps
Age: Age:

Eczema   Rheumatic fever
Age: Age:

Chicken pox
Age:

Scarlet fever
Age:

German measles
Age:

Whooping cough
Age:

Present medication:

Allergies:

Previous illnesses:

Medical
Surgical

Social history:

<u>*Lifestyle*</u>

Smoking:

Do you smoke now? ..... cigarettes ..... cigars ..... pipe .....

If you have stopped smoking:

When did you stop? .... What was the daily maximum smoked then? ......

Have you tried to give up? ....

Have you cut down? (Yes) when? .... and by how many? ....

What is the maximum number per day you have ever smoked? ......

Alcohol:

How much alcohol do you drink per week: *beer:* ....
wine: ....
spirits: ....

Height: What is your height? ....

Weight: What is your weight? ....

Would you say you are *underweight*? ....

Would you say you are *overweight*? ....

Have you lost weight recently? .... How much? ....

Have you gained weight recently? .... How much? ....

Family history

Do you or any of your family or close relatives have or had any of the following:

	Yes	No	Details
Diabetes			
High blood pressure			
Heart attack			
Stroke			
Epilepsy or fit			
Asthma			
Skin disease			
Nervous disorders			
Allergies			
Congenital diseases			
Cancer			
Kidney disease			

Immunisation history:

Please indicate if you have been immunised against the following illnesses, giving details of last immunisation:

German measles
Influenza
Measles
Mumps
Polio
Tetanus
Typhoid
Whooping cough

Women only:

Periods:

At what age did your periods start? ....
                              finish? .... (if relevant)
Are your periods regular?   ....

How long does the period last?   ....

Please indicate your period cycle (how long between periods):   ....

Do you use contraceptives?   –   The Pill
                             –   Intra-uterine coil
                             –   Cap – Diaphragm
                             –   Sheath
                             –   Other methods

If taking the contraceptive pill – for how long have you taken it?   ....

Have you had a cervical smear?   ....

What was the date of the last cervical smear?   ....

Children:

Please list all children that you have had:

Name: ....

Date of birth: ....

Difficulties with pregnancy or birth: ....

Please give details of any miscarriages you may have had:

NEW PATIENT REGISTRATION CARD

Alternatively, the following brief registration card can be completed by the practice nurse at interview.

Surname:
First name:
Address:
Telephone number:
Date of birth:
Date of registration:

Medical history:

Surgical history:

Medication:
Allergies:
Lifestyle:

Health screen:

Height:
Weight:
Blood pressure:
Urinalysis:

Rubella status
Polio status:
Tetanus status:

Action:

Follow-up:

AIDE-MEMOIRE FOR THE PRACTICE NURSE

Medical history

Occupation:
Heart disease:
Kidney/bladder:
Chest/asthma:
Digestive/liver:
Joint/back:
Diabetes/thyroid:
Gynaecological:
Operations:
Past screening procedures:
Allergies:
Medication:

Social/lifestyle

Smoking:
Alcohol:
Exercise:
Diet:
Stress factors:

Present state of health:

Process of the interview – following agreed practice protocol

The basic health screen should include:

- height
- weight $\Big\}$ = body mass index
- blood pressure
- urine test

For female entrants it may be appropriate to check on family planning and cervical smear status.

Discuss lifestyle issues that are disclosed at interview or in the questionnaire.

Identify health concerns and refer appropriately.

Up-date immunisations status.

(Where there are indications for a clinical procedure needing to be undertaken, e.g. family planning or cervical smear test, the patient should be given an appropriate appointment.)

If, on the other hand, it is decided within the practice protocol that such clinical care as family planning or cervical smear testing should be undertaken opportunistically, more time should be allocated to each appointment.

SENIOR CITIZENS

The New Contract proposes higher capitation fees for patients over the age of 75 years, providing that they are assessed annually by a member of the practice team and the patient's well-being recorded.

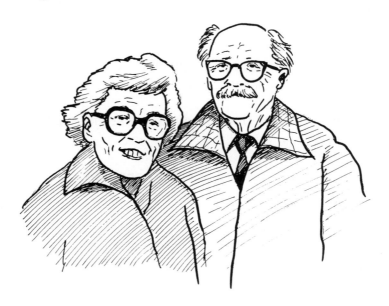

The following check list is a guide:
- Clinical condition
- Mental state
- Special senses including vision and hearing
- Continence
- General function
- Lifestyle
- Social assessment including support
- Hobbies and interests
- Review of medication
- Plan for continuing care

We have been screening the senior citizens of the practice and use the following forms and procedures.

The *aim* of this assessment is to determine the health and social needs of the patient and refer them to the appropriate agency to deal with their needs, e.g. doctor/health visitor and/or voluntary agency.

Forms and procedures:
- identify groups to be screened
- determine who is to screen this group of patients
- determine the staff to be involved and identify their roles
- inform patients well in advance of the proposed assessment using method identified in the case history
- allocate appropriate resources

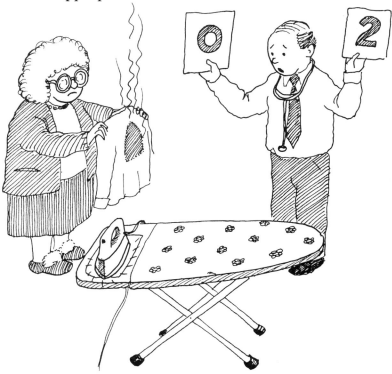

"Marks for technical merit"

QUESTIONNAIRE

Name: Marital status: Sex: DOB:

First names: Doctor:

Address:

Telephone number:

Next of kin   *Chief carer*

Surname: Surname

First names: First names:

Address: Address:

Telephone number: Telephone number:

Relationship: Age: Relationship: Age

Emergency contact

Telephone number:

Housing: Solitude:

Home safety: Regular help:

Social support:

Nursing assessment:

Mobility:

Personal hygiene: Communication:

Special senses: Sight:

                        Hearing:

Feeding: Dentition:

Sleeping:

Mental state: Condition of patient:

Medication:

Diet: Skin:

Bladder: Bowels:

Warmth:

Other help: Urine test:
                 BP:
                 Respiration:

Action required: Medical ⎞
                 Social   ⎬ refer to local agencies
                 Voluntary ⎠

Note

This method of assessing patients in their own home can identify their ability to manage within their own home: security, maintenance and general safety.

ELDERLY AT-RISK REGISTER

The establishment of a manual system at-risk register for the elderly of the practice came about following the visiting of some of our senior citizens in their home setting, and following our 'elderly pop-in afternoon' where a health assessment is carried out and an aspect of health care considered in depth.

The AIM of the register is:

To provide a quick, highly visual detailed information card of those patients considered to be 'at-risk'.

Factors to consider when setting up an elderly at-risk register:

1. Accessibility of the information to all parties concerned
2. Easy to understand
3. Readily capable of being updated.

ESSENTIAL INFORMATION

Name: Date of birth:
Address:

Telephone number: Means of access:
Next of kin: Name:
                                   Address:
                                   Telephone number:

Problems: Medical problems
                                   Medication
Support/Services
Medical:

Social:

Date of assessment:

Screening programme for the elderly: Case history

The following case history identifies the methods that can be adopted to screen this client group.

Experience of one practice

A practice of 12 000 population had 874 patients over the age of 75 years identified on a computer printout.

A series of meetings with all members of the primary health care team were held over working lunches at the practice, with each patient on the list being discussed and identified. All patients were eliminated who were known to have services appropriate to their needs, or whose general health and well-being was satisfactory, and it was known no services were required.

The members of the primary care team failed to identify 156 patients as being known to them.

The records of these patients were pulled; 6 of whom were found to be on regular medication and known to the practice, this left 150 patients to be assessed. A health questionnaire was written and approved by all members of the team and this was used in the following way, divided into 3 equal groups.

– _Group 1:_ This group was visited by the district nurse or health visitor.

– _Group 2:_ The practice invited groups of 15 to attend the surgery on an afternoon to discuss health matters with the practice nurses and health visitor.

– _Group 3:_ The questionnaire used for the other two groups was posted to each patient and they were asked to kindly complete it and return it to the practice in the stamped and addressed envelope enclosed with the questionnaire.

The greatest success was by personal contact and in _all_ groups the identified problems were 90% related to social issues and 10% to health care.

Although the greatest response was achieved by personal contact this is very costly in terms of professional time and the outcomes to identify health care needs did not justify this method of contact.

As a quick check the table shows what should be carried out in the various groups and clinics:

target groups	HT	WT	BP	peak flow	urine	hear	sight	cx smear
elderly		✔	✔		✔	✔	✔	
new patients	✔	✔	✔	✔	✔			
well woman	✔	✔	✔	✔	✔			✔
well man	✔	✔	✔	✔	✔			
pre-conceptual	✔	✔	✔		✔			✔
pre-retirement	✔	✔	✔	✔	✔	✔	✔	
young adults F	✔	✔	✔	✔	✔			✔
M	✔	✔	✔	✔	✔			

breast exam	testicular self: exam	ECG	diet	alcohol	smoking	relations	exer.	Hb	lipids
			✔	✔	✔	✔		✔	
			✔	✔	✔				
✔			✔	✔	✔	✔	✔	✔	
	✔	✔	✔	✔	✔	✔	✔	✔	✔
✔			✔	✔	✔	✔	✔		–
			✔	✔	✔	✔	✔		
✔	✔		✔✔	✔✔	✔✔	✔✔	✔✔		

FLOW CHARTS

It is helpful for the practice to produce simple flow charts to show what actions should be taken when an abnormality is detected. Examples for hypertension and cervical smears are shown.

Hypertension

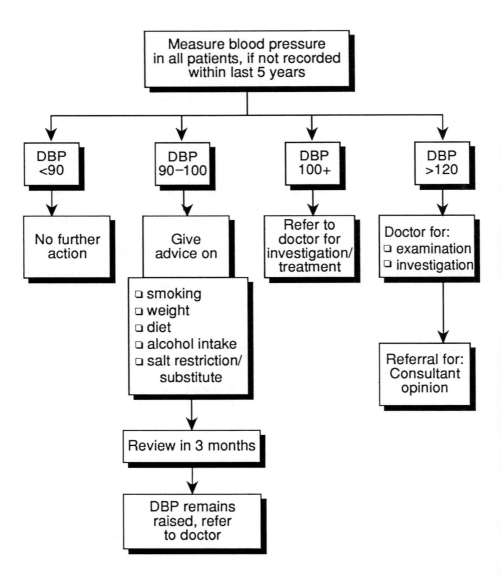

Cervical Smears

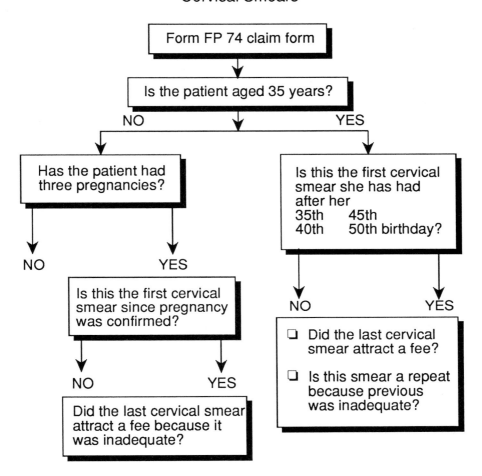

1. 'First cervical smear' means
   first cervical smear performed
   by any agency including
   general practitioner.

2. Repeat fees are not paid for
   any cervical smear taken
   as part of a course of treatment.

3. Claims must be submitted
   within 6 months of taking
   the cervical smear.

Chapter 3

TRAINING

Effective screening is a specialised procedure which should be undertaken by staff who have a clear understanding of the importance of the screening exercise and have been trained to fulfil their roles.

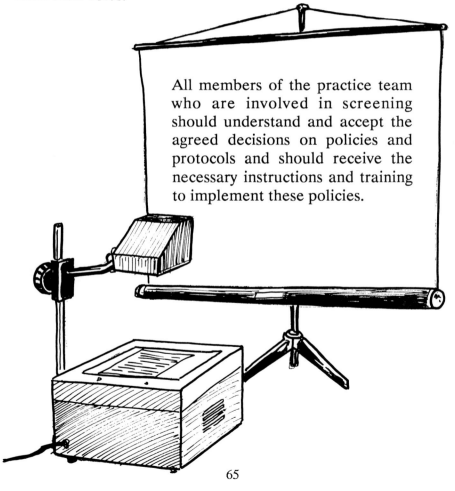

All members of the practice team who are involved in screening should understand and accept the agreed decisions on policies and protocols and should receive the necessary instructions and training to implement these policies.

Each member of the practice team who is clearly involved in screening procedures should have his/her roles clearly identified in their job descriptions and appropriate training programmes implemented.

TRAINING PROGRAMMES

There are two types of training programmes:

1. *In-service*

   Members of the screening team can be trained within the practice to fulfil their identified roles.

   – clerical support by the practice administrator
   – clinical procedures by the general practitioner and/or senior practice nurse within the practice

2. *Outside courses*

   Courses organised by various local and national bodies who can train specialist members of the team, e.g. doctors and practice nurses

It is best to consider possibilities before embarking on a training programme:

– *Who should be trained?* – all the practice team require 'training' but for some it should be more detailed; the numbers involved will influence the type of exercise.

– *What training?* – it should include motivation, improvement of attitude, provision of information, knowledge, teaching skills and procedures.

- *Where?* – an early decision has to be taken whether some, if any, of the practice team should be sent on outside courses, bearing in mind the need for absence cover, or whether an in-service programme would be more appropriate.

Training courses could be organised through the general practitioner course tutor in each district.

- *When?* – an in-service programme has to be arranged outside normal working hours, either evenings or at weekends.

- *Who to teach* – most aspects can be undertaken by members of the team, but it may be felt that some outsiders with experience might be better, such as a GP who has experience in his/her own practice, or practice manager, senior practice nurse, or a management consultant.

In-service training programmes

For such a programme to be undertaken, one member of the team should be appointed as the organiser. This person will need to decide on:

- aims and objectives of the programme
- content and methods of teaching
- who is to do the teaching
- teaching programme
- assessment and evaluation

Matters of particular importance that have to be addressed are:

- legal and ethical responsibilities of all staff involved

- patient's consent
- confidentiality

The doctors are covered by their Medical Defence Organisation and the nurses by the Royal College of Nursing or the Medical Defence Union. Ultimate responsibility must rest with the senior member of the team, who will be the doctor. If, however, the doctor delegates the responsibility to the practice nurse, and the nurse accepts then she is bound by the code of professional conduct of the United Kingdom central council for nurses, midwives and health visitors.

In-service training education programmes

1. General introduction about the screening programme to be undertaken. (It is suggested you identify the members of the practice team who will be the key workers for specific screening programmes.)

2. The client group involved.

3. The aims and objectives of the programme

Practical administrative duties should form part of normal clerical day duties:

- to pull the records
- complete necessary documentation
- enter screening programme in the patient's record
- follow-up defaulters (see page 21)

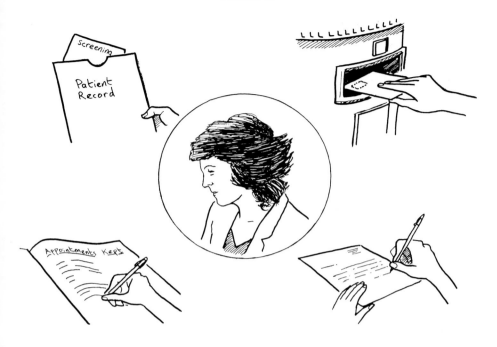

Role of the key worker

The key worker is responsible for the organisation of specific screening programmes, to ensure:

- records are available
- appointments sent
- attendance recorded in liaison with professional staff
- defaulters are followed up

Professional staff

This programme can be undertaken either by the doctor or the senior nurse in the practice or health centre who holds the necessary qualifications.

It is proposed to use the well-woman screening programme as an example of in-service training.

- taking a history
- explanation of the procedure
- height
- weight
- blood pressure
- urinalysis
- abdominal examination
- pelvic examination
- cervical smear
- breast care
- breast examination
- health promotion
- referral of abnormal findings

AN EXAMPLE OF A PRACTICE PROTOCOL FOR CERVICAL SMEAR

Aim
Each sexually active woman in the practice is to be offered a cervical smear every three years unless otherwise indicated by the patient's history, or the cytologist's recommendations.

Role of the clerical records clerk
Before the test, the medical records of the woman are pulled and the necessary forms are completed.

If the patient/client is to be called for a cervical smear test the appropriate letter is sent and signed either by the doctor, practice nurse or practice administrator.

Role of the practice nurse
- check date of last cervical smear
- check date of last menstrual period and enquire if any changes or worries

---

- check if there has been any:
    post-menopausal bleeding
    post-coital bleeding
    inter-menstrual bleeding
- check contraception
- check obstetric history
- determine whether the woman has any vaginal, bladder, or coitus symptoms or problems
- review medical record and patient's history if any significant past infections (pelvic inflammatory diseases, genital warts, herpes, chlamydia infection)
- smoking history
- general well-being of patient
- check weight
- check blood pressure
- health promotion as appropriate
- abdominal examination
- vulval examination
- high vaginal swab if appropriate
- cervical smear noting condition of the cervix
- bi-manual pelvic examination
- answer any queries, worries and talk through findings and how patient will receive result of smear test
- re-call patient or refer as appropriate

Administration with clerical and secretarial support
The practice nurse is responsible for ensuring that those patients of the practice who are eligible for a cervical smear are invited at least twice for this procedure to be undertaken.

If the patienty fails to respond to a second invitation, he/she is referred to the doctor for follow-up.

The practice nurse is also responsible for operating a call and re-call system and notifying the patients of their results, and for ensuring that results are made available to the practice team and entered on the practice computer.

The practice will agree, as a matter of practice protocol, who will sign the various letters relating to cervical smearing.

The protocol will be reviewed in one year.

Outside courses

There is a growing number of courses and ways in which screening can be carried out and health promoted. There follow some examples of courses with which we are familiar and in which we have participated.

Training programmes

The following is the outline curriculum approved by the English National Board which offers a framework for innovation and adaptation to meet the changing needs of practice nurses or treatment room nurses.

Aim: To prepare the practice nurse to work as a member of the primary health care team, confident and competent to provide skilled nursing care within the health centre or practice setting.

Objectives: To enable the practice nurse to:

a)   review and broaden existing professional knowledge and skills and acquire new learning appropriate to her role.

b)   increase knowledge and understanding of the role and responsibilities of other members of the primary health care team and of any other agencies with whom the nurse must liaise and communicate.

c)   increase awareness of factors known to influence interpersonal communications and to develop skills in establishing and maintaining effective communications.

Course guidelines: Course content will be based on three areas of study:

a) professional role development
b) procedures and techniques to be used in the treatment room/health centre
c) management of the treatment room/health centre

Professional role development:

a) Role and function: The role and function of practice nurses in general, with particular attention to the situation in which the individual nurse is working

b) The primary health care team concept: The philosophy of primary health care; the organisation of general practice and community nursing; the role and function of individual team members and of members of agencies with whom the nurse will expect to be in regular contact.

c) Nursing intervention: Application of the nursing process approach to the observation and care of patients/clients suffering from conditions met within the treatment room.

d) Responsibility and accountability: The nurse's professional responsibility and accountability for her own standards of care and for keeping up to date with changing trends in medical and nursing practice; legal and ethical aspects of role performance; the boundaries of decision making; access to and use of local learning resources.

e) Recording and reporting: The principles of accurate recording and reporting; the use and storage of records and effective use of local record systems.

f) Drug management: The safe administration and storage of drugs; the use and purpose of the drug tariff book.

g) Equipment: The care and maintenance of equipment in the treatment room.

h) Communications: Establishing and maintaining relationships with patients, colleagues and employers/managers; an introduction to methods and techniques of counselling and advising others; recognising and using lines of communication and accountability and methods of liaison and co-operation.

i) Patient teaching/health education: An introduction to the basic principles of patient teaching/health education and their application is one-to-one teaching situations; knowledge of organisations involved in health education and how to obtain and use available resources.

j) Identifying the needs of special groups: Signs of family violence, abuse and/or neglect – knowledge of local policy and procedures, ethnic minority groups, disabled persons.

Procedures, techniques and knowledge required for working in the treatment room:

a) The collection, handling and transportation of laboratory specimens, including blood samples; vene- puncture.

b) Electrocardiography, the care, maintenance and use of the electrocardiograph machine.

c) Immunisation, vaccination of children, adults and travellers; up to date knowledge of WHO recommendations with regard to travellers; other injections and vaccines; de-sensitizing procedures.

d) Knowledge of screening procedures, including blood pressure, cervical cytology, examination of the breast, skin testing, vitalography, peak flow meter.

e) Preparation of the eye for examination; common eye treatments and removal of foreign bodies.

f) Examination and common treatments of the ear; use of the auriscope; ear syringing.

g) Application of special dressings and bandages.

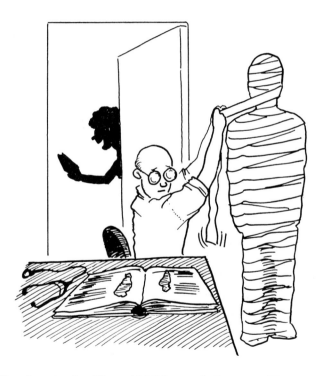

"Ah, there's the First Aid Manual, Doctor. Now where did I leave my book on Egyptology?"

h)   Application of surgical collars and other orthopaedic appliances.

i)   Family planning: basic knowledge of various methods of contraception, basic information about sterilization, termination of pregnancy, infertility. For those nurses who are involved in family planning it is recommended that they attend the English National Board Course 900.

j)   First aid and management of emergencies such as:
     – cardiac arrest
     – injuries – sprains, fractures, wounds
     – haemorrhage
     – anaphylactic shock
     – inhalation of foreign bodies, ingestion of poisonous substances
     – burns and scalds
     – fainting

k)   Drugs: controlled drugs – use and misuse; pharmacology of common drugs; drugs commonly used in general practice; drug reactions and interactions including over-dosage of drugs.

l)   Recognition and treatment of simple skin conditions.

m)   Knowledge of, and nursing care of, minor ailments and simple medical conditions, upper respiratory tract infections, urinary tract infections, gastroenteritis.

Practice management and administration:
a)   The use and function of reception and appointment systems.

b) Structure and function of the family practitioner committee, procedure for claiming fees and allowances.

c) The use and function of age/sex and observation registers.

d) The use of computers in general practice.

e) Health and welfare of personnel; implications of the Health and Safety at Work Act.

f) Conditions of service.

g) Planning the layout of a treatment room in liaison with the architect.

Learn how to help people stop smoking

A training opportunity for health and welfare workers in hospitals, community, industry and commerce.

A one day training course is offered which covers the following aspects of helping people to stop smoking:

− Encouraging people to stop
− How to set up and run support groups
− Information on smoking and health
− Practical aspects of stopping smoking
− Helping people to remain non-smokers

Courses are held regularly at venues around the country. Details and application form from:

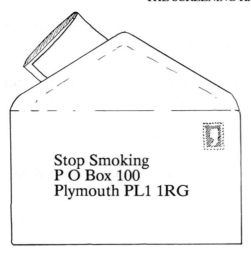

Stop Smoking
P O Box 100
Plymouth PL1 1RG

Anticipatory Care in General Practice (ACT)

ACT began in 1985 as a working group of general practitioners and practice nurses seeking ways to reduce the incidence of heart disease through prevention in primary care. ACT activities, group newsletter and bulletin are regularly sent to members. Those interested in the work of the group or in joining should contact:

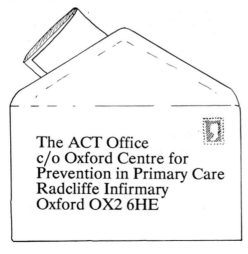

The ACT Office
c/o Oxford Centre for
Prevention in Primary Care
Radcliffe Infirmary
Oxford OX2 6HE

Hypertension

Training days for practice nurses are organised in Birmingham on behalf of the British Hypertension Society by Dr. G.R. Beevers. For information on courses, contact Dr. Beevers' secretary at:

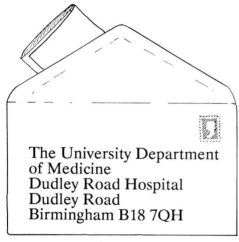

The University Department
of Medicine
Dudley Road Hospital
Dudley Road
Birmingham B18 7QH

Practice Nurse programmes

Continuing education programme for practice nurses which includes lectures, group work and exercises designed to improve the nurse's knowledge, attitudes and skills for her work and to her patients.

Continuing education units system enables practice nurses to record and monitor their own training progress.

The first module covers such topics as:

− Practice organisation
− First aid and emergencies

- Health promotion and the prevention of heart disease
- The management of hypertension, asthma and diabetes
- Communication skills
- The development of practice nursing

For further details:

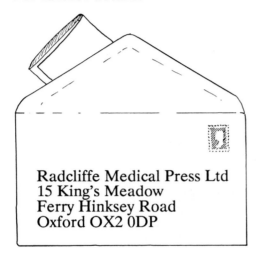

Radcliffe Medical Press Ltd
15 King's Meadow
Ferry Hinksey Road
Oxford OX2 0DP

Distance learning

English National Board for Nursing, Midwifery and Health Visiting: Distance Learning Packages (funded by government).

Health Promotion is the first of what will be a continuing series especially designed to meet the needs of practice nurses.

The *First Module* begins by explaining how the course originators see distance learning's place in the professional development of the practice nurse, and gives guidance on what, for most users, will be a new style of learning:

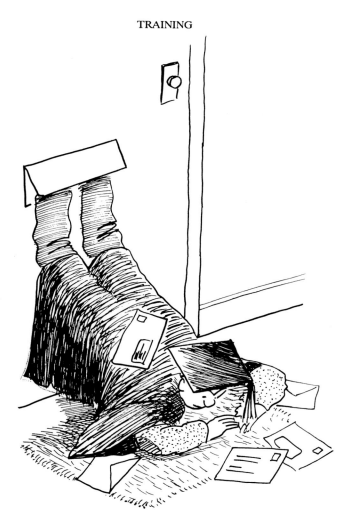

The correspondence course arrives

- how to choose from the material according to need, and
- how to work through selected topics individually or with others.

A framework for the series is then provided by a detailed exploration of:

- Health promotion
- Health education
- The role of the primary health care team
- Developing teamwork
- The organisation of care.

The *Second Module* is the first of a series of clinical updates and deals with cervical screening:

- Why carry out screening?
- Assessment of need
- Planning of care
- Implementation of care
- Evaluation of care

Details from:

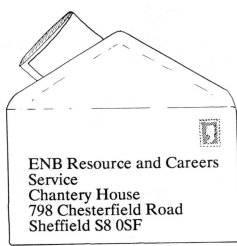

ENB Resource and Careers
Service
Chantery House
798 Chesterfield Road
Sheffield S8 0SF

Distance learning package for practice nurses

Nurses have a code of professional conduct produced by the United Kingdom Central Council for Nurses, Midwifery and Health Visiting (UKCC) which clearly indicates the nurses responsibilities for practice.

The introduction to the code states:

'Each registered nurse, midwife or health visitor shall act, at all times, in such a good manner as to justify public trust and confidence, to uphold and enhance the good standing and reputation of the profession, to serve the interest of society, and above all to safeguard the interests of individual patients and clients.

'Each registered nurse, midwife and health visitor is accountable for his or her practice . . . '

There are fourteen items listed in the code but the two most relevant to education and training are:

3. 'Take every reasonable opportunity to maintain and improve professional knowledge and competence

4. Acknowledge any limitations of competence and refuse in such cases to accept delegated functions without first having received instruction in regard to those functions and having been assessed as competent.'

The distance learning package entitled 'Health Promotion in Primary Health Care' has been specifically designed for practice nurses.

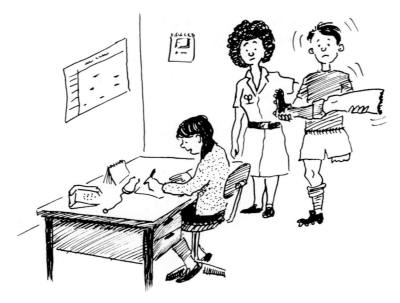

"I'm very busy, Sister. Just put a stitch in that for me please."

Health Promotion Booklet Summary

The consumer perspective:
- highlights new thinking about primary health care. This section contains an audio tape of two BBC radio programmes in the Seven Ages of Health series. It illustrates the needs of the consumer as expressed by the consumer and talks about the role of the practice nurse in relation to the people she cares for. This topic should help the practice nurse to:

  - assess how far the practice policies meet the needs of the people who use the health services

  - review how well she/he listens to a major consumer group within the practice

- assess opportunities for extending work with groups of health service users within the practice

- review the ways in which the practice can promote health alongside medicine and nursing.

Health promotion and health education:
- defines and explores the meaning of the terms health promotion and health education. A wide range of activities fall under the umbrella of health promotion, decisions need to be made using the decision process in order to help the practice nurse decide which topics are appropriate for her to be involved in. The topic should help the nurse to:

- consider some of the different meanings of health
- identify important influences on health and illness
- be aware of factors which affect an individual's decision about health and illness
- define health promotion and the role of health education within it
- identify her/his own learning needs in relation to health promotion
- review the health promotion activities already being undertaken in the practice
- review the health promotion activities that the practice nurse is undertaking or would like to undertake
- draw up a practice profile in order to access health education needs of different targetted groups

The skills of health education:
- examines the opportunities for health education with individuals and small groups. It describes the skills needed by the practice nurse in her/his role as health educator and suggests ways of assessing developing those skills. This topic should help the practice nurse to:

- assess his/her skill in communicating with individuals
- plan, undertake and review one-to-one health education
- make the most of unplanned opportunities for health education
- help people change their health behaviour
- think about opportunities for group work if appropriate

Who's involved in primary health care:
- investigates the role of individuals within the team and the need for a team approach. Knowing what members of the primary health care team and other agencies do is a vital first step towards forming links with other team members which can only improve working together. This topic should help the practice nurse to:

  - understand the roles of practice-based primary health care team members
  - review reception procedures as the first point of contact for users
  - describe the roles of other agencies involved
  - identify ways in which these bodies could be of help in the practice nurse's work and plan how to improve communication with them
  - identify how the membership of primary health care teams may differ, according to the user's needs and circumstances

Developing teamwork:
- looks at the common characteristics of teams. It looks at how primary health care teams develop and how the obstacles which often get in the way of effective teamwork can be overcome. This topic should help the nurse to:

- understand that caring for people and patients involves other members of the practice
- realise that primary health care teams do not always work well together and much effort needs to be made to help teams to work together
- realise that the team may be more effective if it is understood what makes teams work well together and what makes teams fail

Organisation of care:
- highlights the need for individual and team objectives, so everyone knows what they are aiming for and can evaluate if they are achieving their objectives. Protocols are discussed as a way of co-ordinating shared care. The topic should help the nurse to:

  - understand the importance of setting aims and objectives for her/his work
  - define objectives for his/her work and how to use these as a basis of evaluation
  - participate in objective setting with other members of the primary health care team
  - promote the advantages of team meetings
  - understand the contributions made by nursing to primary health care, and differentiate them from the contributions of other professionals
  - work with colleagues on drawing up protocols to co-ordinate care that is shared

Cervical Screening Booklet Summary

This part of the learning package deals with a skill. The skill is that of taking a cervical smear. The opportunity is taken at the same time of considering wider implications of how women coming forward for a cervical smear feel, what the nurse can do to provide an efficient all round programme of care and how to evaluate the care given.

Offering a smear test and encouraging women to have this screening procedure undertaken is an area in which practice nurses have a major role to play in health promotion and health education. The topic should help the nurse to:

- understand the need for an organised screening programme
- identify who should be screened
- identify the skills needed to be able to carry out screening
- communicate clearly and understand the concerns of the women having the test
- gain an understanding of aetiology and epidemiological background of cervical cancer
- evaluate the care the nurse is providing

Marie Curie Foundation

The Marie Curie Foundation with funding from the Department of Health has recently begun a 3-year programme of cancer screening courses for practice nurses.

Each course comprises the 2-day modules held on consecutive weeks, with a follow-up day 6 months later, and teaches participants breast and pelvic examination and how to take a cervical smear.

Courses are held through the United Kingdom and are facilitated by an experienced practice nurse.

For further details:

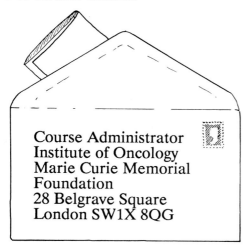

Course Administrator
Institute of Oncology
Marie Curie Memorial
Foundation
28 Belgrave Square
London SW1X 8QG

The Marie Curie Memorial Foundation Institute of Oncology
Breast and Cervical Screening Course for Practice Nurses

Outline curriculum

Aim: To provide trained nurses (initially practice nurses) with
the appropriate knowledge and skills to screen women for
breast and cervical cancer.

Objectives: At the end of the course the nurse will:

– understand the relevant normal anatomy, physiology and
  cytopathology of the pelvis and breast including associated
  structures
– recognise the value of a criterion for early detection of
  breast and cervical cancer
– appreciate the implications of actual screening for these two
  conditions

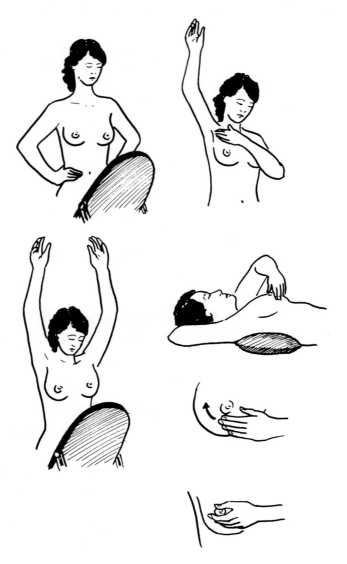

- understand the effect of disease on these two sites and the resulting abnormal pathology
- establish or extend good communications skills to facilitate relationships with both clients and colleagues

- extend skills in taking the client's history in the context of cervical and breast screening
- demonstrate skills to support and counsel clients and those close to them (whether families or friends) to help them cope with the physical and psychological impact of breast and cervical screening
- perceive and initiate the health education role with clients

Cervical screening:
- demonstrate competence to carry out pelvic and cervical examinations
- demonstrate competence to obtain a cervical smear from a variety of women
- demonstrate the ability to prepare a good slide of the cervical smear and despatch it appropriately
- be aware of the need for safe practice in the handling of body fluids
- utilise current research and statutory information to contribute to an efficient cervical screening programme
- collaborate with statutory and voluntary organisations to provide the best care for clients

Breast screening:
- recognise the features of a normal, healthy breast with adjacent structures
- be competent to detect obvious abnormalities in the breast
- demonstrate the ability to systematically examine the breast in a variety of women
- be able to teach women breast self-awareness and examination as appropriate
- appreciate the use of technology to confirm breast abnormalities

Women's National Cancer Control Campaign (WNCCC)

The WNCCC is a registered charity primarily concerned with the prevention and early detection of cancer in women.

The latest video – *Ray of Hope* – demonstrates the technique of mammography and describes the government's breast screening programme. The video shows a woman undertaking breast self-examination and describes the kind of changes and symptoms which might indicate the presence of breast cancer, or the more common benign breast diseases. (The video runs for 22 minutes.)

The video can be purchased or hired.

Further information from:

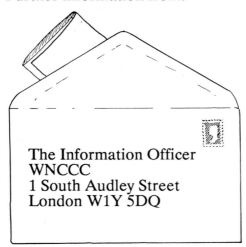

The Information Officer
WNCCC
1 South Audley Street
London W1Y 5DQ

Open University

The *Open University's* Department of Health and Social Welfare provides a range of study packs for individual and group use.

'Coronary Heart Disease: Reducing the Risk' is a study pack developed in association with the Health Education Authority.

The course aims to help primary health care workers, including practice nurses, GPs, health visitors, district nurses, practice managers and receptionists to:

- become informed about the issues involved in coronary heart disease risk reduction

- review evidence for the risk factors of coronary heart disease and the effectiveness of interventions to lower them

- develop their approach to note assessment and management, and the special records that such work requires

- make use of community resources and consider opportunities they have to contribute to inter-community-based health promotion initiatives.

For information:

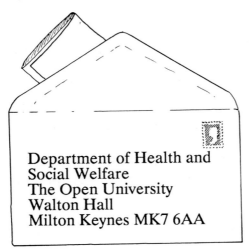

Department of Health and
Social Welfare
The Open University
Walton Hall
Milton Keynes MK7 6AA

Chapter 4

RESOURCES

For screening to be effective, attention must be paid to providing the necessary resources.

These can be examined under 4 headings:

- Manpower/personnel
- Accommodation
- Equipment
- Disposables

MANPOWER/PERSONNEL

In planning screening it is necessary to identify the tasks of individual team members.

- *Administrative*
  Someone has to be responsible for organising the clinic or process. This is most likely to be the practice manager or nurse, but it can be anyone, one of the doctors or secretaries. Whoever it is, she (or he) must set out on paper the steps involved.

- *Secretarial*
  The secretariat will have the task of selecting the patients to be screened; checking addresses (possibly 1 in 4 may have changed from the original when the patient registered); sending out appointments; and arranging for confirmation.

– *Reception staff*

Will be on hand to receive the patients on the correct day and time and organise a smooth patient-flow, also checking and arranging for follow-up for patients to be informed of results and making further appointments.

– *Professional staff*

Are those who will undertake the screening. These will be practice nurses, or other professional personnel.

– *Doctors*

One, or more, of the general practitioners should be present during the screening and be available to provide advice and support, such as dealing with any major abnormalities discovered (rarely) or in assisting in any problems that may occur, such as reactions to venepuncture, injections, difficulties with cervical smears, interpreting ECGs and dealing with difficult patients.

ACCOMODATION

The accommodation that will be required includes that for:
– waiting area
– interview
– examination
– tests/investigations

Some of these may be combined, but have to be detailed in advance.

All practice premises are busy and occupied and availability must be planned and secured well in advance, but only once the frequency and duration of the clinics have been determined.

Ground floor accommodation has to be reserved for elderly, handicapped and mothers and babies.

Obviously there has to be space to include all the facilities that may be required, including any for emergency resuscitation.

A check list is useful.

EQUIPMENT

A check list must include basic and special items of equipment:

Basic
    Couch
    Desk
    Chairs
    Scales
        – adult
        – children
    Height measure
    Baby length measure
    Eye vision charts
    Urine testing equipment
    Sterilisers (Hotair/autoclave) Refer to *A code of practice for sterilisation of instruments and control of cross infection* (1989) British Medical Association
    Speculae (vaginal)
    Sphygmomanometer
    Stethoscope
    Tape measure
    Angle-poise lamp
    Trolley
    Microscope

Specific
Peak flow meter
Vitalograph
ECG
Sonic aid
Auroscope

Equipment for child development available from:

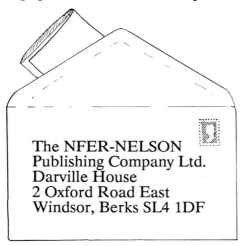

The NFER-NELSON
Publishing Company Ltd.
Darville House
2 Oxford Road East
Windsor, Berks SL4 1DF

Disposables

These have become modern medical essentials, their choice
and selection is largely personal:

– tissues
– couch sheets
– wipes
– latex gloves
– protective clothing
– chemical reagents

ORGANISATION

To summarise, it is essential to plan ahead and to adhere to allocated timing. This should be done by:

- arranging appointments suitable for the practice and patients

- organising use of consulting and other rooms

- ensuring availability of equipment

- staff knowing their individual roles with prior in-service and pilot trials

- reception staff organising patient flow and arranging for follow-up of non-attender

CHECK-LIST OF EQUIPMENT

	elderly	new patient	well women	well men
couch	✔	✔	✔	✔
desk	✔	✔	✔	✔
chairs	✔	✔	✔	✔
trolley	✔	✔	✔	✔
scales: adult	✔	✔	✔	✔
: children		✔		
height measure : adult		✔		
: baby		✔		
urine testing:	✔	✔	✔	✔
sphygmoma-nometer	✔	✔	✔	✔
stethoscope	✔	✔	✔	✔
tape measure				
speculae assorted			✔	
sterilizer			✔	
sonic aid				
peak flow/ vitalograph		✔		✔
ECG				✔
eye charts	✔			
auroscope	✔			

pre-conceptual	young adult M	F	child surveillance	ante-natal	pre-retirement
✔	✔			✔	✔
✔	✔			✔	✔
✔	✔			✔	✔
✔	✔			✔	✔
✔	✔	✔	specialist equipment	✔	✔
✔	✔	✔		✔	✔
✔	✔	✔		✔	✔
✔	✔	✔		✔	✔
✔		✔		✔	✔
✔		✔		✔	
				✔	
	✔	✔			
					✔
					✔
					✔

Chapter 5

COSTS

Screening is expensive in time and money, and careful budgeting, administration and organisation are necessary to ensure that it is cost effective and beneficial to providers as well as consumers. Ultimately, it is the practice and the National Health Service, through the Family Practitioner Committee, who are the providers, and who have to meet costs and supply the resources. Assurance of evidence of benefits to public and personal health is difficult to obtain, but a built-in audit review system should be incorporated and results published for critical examination.

Although there is some reimbursement from the Family Practitioner Committee for procedures that attract item of service payments, much of the cost is and will be borne by the practice.

EXPENDITURE COSTS

Itemisation of expenditure should be broad and detailed if proper accounting is to be achieved. It covers many areas:

Practice
- administration and organisation
- staff
- equipment
- maintenance

Patients
- earning loss
- travel
- other incidentals

ADMINISTRATION AND ORGANISATION

Excluding the opportunistic screening that is part of the consultation process, planning should assume that a screening clinic will last for 3 hours, with 20-minute patient consultations, or 9–10 persons being seen.

Further, we have found that it takes up to 2 hours of staff time to call and process invitations to these 9–10 patients.

Expenditure includes checking records, computer use (if available), stationery, postage and phone calls.

STAFF

Staff includes secretarial, receptionist and nursing input, with approximate rates from £3 to £7 per hour. In addition, there may have to be payments for training.

EQUIPMENT

The outlay of equipment will depend on the type and extent of screening programme planned. Standard equipment such as sphygmomanometers, peak flow meters, height and weight measures will be available, but electrocardiograms, audiometers, tonometers and machines for biochemical measurements may need to be purchased or written down in the expenditure.

A significant cost will be for *disposables*, such as examination gloves, couch sheets and towels, urine testing equipment and that for cervical cytology.

MAINTENANCE

Maintenance costs have to be included and will relate to the amount of time involved. Items for inclusion are cleaning, heat, light, water, repairs and other incidentals.

INCOME GENERATION

Reimbursement of staff, say, is at a rate of 70%, but the practice still has to pay 30%.

New income will come through claims for:

− *cervical cytology* (smears), but only within the current term of service, i.e. in over 35-year-old women, and only one every 5 years. Target payments will be introduced with the new GP contract.

− *family planning.*

− *immunisation* − updating for tetanus and poliomyelitis.

− *special clinics* − under the '1990 Contract' general practitioners will be carrying out health promotion clinics for well persons, elderly observation, child development and minor operations. Fees for these surgeries have not yet been identified.

Case history*

AIM:

To screen nine well women of the practice in a 3-hour clinic – 20 minutes per patient

STAFF INVOLVED:

Administrative and clerical:
- identify clients
- invite clients
- arrange appointments
- pull records
- complete necessary documents for client
- follow-up defaulters

Total time 2 hours costed at clerical officer grade £3.50 per hour.

Nursing:

3 hour session including:
- preparation of the equipment
- preparation of the clinic
- documentation of patients' records
- safe disposal of specimens
- safe disposal of clinical waste
- decontamination and sterilisation of equipment

RGN G grade £7.10 average per hour

Specific expenditure:
- cleaning
- heat
- light
- maintenance

Average cost per clinic £2.50

* Prices correct at time of going to press

Specific items:
Cost of disposable equipment

- disposable speculae 75p
- disposable latex gloves 8p per glove
- plastic apron 25p
- cytobrushes 18–20p each
- slides, fixative, transport containers, spatulae are currently provided by most Health Authorities

The cost of such a clinic to the practice will be about £45 and this does not include any doctor's time which is estimated at £30 per hour.

APPENDIX – Urine Testing Equipment*

- Multistix 10 SG reagent strips (recommended retail price excluding VAT = bottle × 100 strips £25.25) for:
    - pH
    - Protein
    - Glucose
    - Ketones
    - Bilirubin
    - Blood
    - Nitrite
    - Urobilinogen
    - Specific gravity
    - Leukocytes
- N-Labstix Reagent strips (recommended retail price excluding VAT = bottle × 100 strips £18.55) for:
    - pH
    - Protein
    - Glucose
    - Ketones
    - Blood
    - Nitrite
- Hema-Combistix Reagent strips (recommended retail price excluding VAT = bottle × 50 strips £8.68) for:
    - pH
    - Protein
    - Glucose
    - Blood
- Uristix Reagent strips (recommended retail price excluding VAT = bottle × 50 strips £5.44) for:
    - Protein
    - Glucose
- Albostix Reagent strips (F.P.10 prescribable. Recommended retail price excluding VAT = bottle × 50 strips £3.51) for:
    - Protein
- Diastix Reagent strips (F.P.10 prescribable. Recommended retail price excluding VAT = bottle × 50 strips £2.55) for:
    - Glucose (semi-quantitative)

* Prices correct at time of going to press

Chapter 6

EVALUATION

The screening exercise must be subjected to the same critical and rigorous examination and evaluation as any other procedure in medicine. There have to be regular 'audits' or reviews and analyses of achievements in meeting goals and checks on organisation and administration.

Therefore, it is advisable that such checks and audits should be incorporated into every screening programme. It is wasteful and less than useful for a practice to become involved in screening merely because it is fashionable and because other local practices are carrying it out. Screening is expensive in time, effort and money, and there has to be evidence that it is well rewarded in benefits for all involved.

BASIC QUESTIONS

There are some basic questions that apply to all screening programmes.

- How many of the target groups have attended and what responses have there been in various methods of invitation? What reasons for non-attendance?

- How reliable are the methods and systems of screening?

- How many 'abnormalities' have been detected and how important and significant are they?

- What findings on follow-up? For example, have smokers given up smoking and have heavy drinkers cut down or abstained? Has there been compliance in dieting and in following therapeutic regimes?

- What have been the views of consumers? What opinions on the concept of screening? How convenient the arrangements? What reactions and responses to advice given?

ATTENDANCE RATES

There are groups of 'attenders' and 'non-attenders'. There are the *possibles* whose names appear in the age–sex register, and there are the *invitees* who are actually invited to come to the screening sessions.

- *possibles*: it is more important to note the proportions of all those at-risk who attend than of the invitees. However, the age–sex register, no matter how enthusiastically it is kept, has errors. In many practices more than 1 in 10 of addresses will be wrong because patients do not inform when they move within the practice area and women marry and do not inform of their married names.

- *invitees*: provided that with careful preparation the screening exercise has been publicised, the timing of sessions is convenient and that patients are invited a month or so beforehand, then a high, up to 90%, attendance can be achieved. Non-attenders should be telephoned the next day and offered another appointment. It may be considered appropriate to telephone the day before the session to check.

METHODS OF SCREENING

Periodic checks should be made that the methods used to measure indices, such as blood pressure, pulmonary function, urinalysis, and even height and weight (with or without clothes and shoes!) are comparable and validated between the nurses and doctors taking part. With more sophisticated methods, such as cervical smears and blood cholesterol measurements, then even more care has to be taken to ensure reliability.

ABNORMALITIES

The aim of the screening process is to pick out 'abnormalities' that can be treated or managed to prevent problems in the future.

This laudable objective is fine providing that there is prior agreement on what is an 'abnormality'.

Thus, it is essential that 'high blood pressure' should be defined, the method of taking it reliable and that it should not be diagnosed on a single reading. Similar reasoning applies to interpretation of blood sugar and cholesterol levels.

Therefore it is likely that the screening will lead to a number of patients having to attend more times in order to decide on the meaning and significance of certain findings, above all, to ensure that long-term advice and treatment should not be undertaken in persons with 'normal abnormalities'.

The record system used must make it possible to see the numbers of abnormalities detailed at a glance, to see who they are, what follow-up has been carried out, and what final outcome.

FOLLOW-UP

As noted, the screening exercise is not a one-off procedure. It is the opportunity to see and examine the patient, to check on measurable indices and to enquire on lifestyle. Those with possible abnormal or equivocal findings have to be seen and assessed again and again to decide on significance of abnormality and on response to treatment, if this has been instituted.

Where risky lifestyles have been detected, then patients must be helped to correct them, i.e. smokers to be helped in stopping, heavy drinkers to control the habit, the overweight to diet and reduce weight and the over-stressed to resolve their fears and anxieties.

Screening can cause more work in the immediate future but, hopefully, it will lead to better health and less work for the practice long-term.

Again an accurate and effective record system is essential to ensure satisfactory results on follow-up.

PATIENTS' VIEWS

Screening primarily is for the benefit of patients. Ideally this message should be made through the practice system of communication. Ideally, also, the scheme works best if organised in consultation and collaboration with a 'patients' group'. Where this does not exist, and in only few practices are there active patient groups, then an *ad hoc* planning group with 2 or 3 invited patients should be created in the early stages to discuss matters, such as publicity and information, timing of sessions, the tests and examinations, reporting results and follow-up.

CRITERIA FOR SUCCESS/NON-SUCCESS

Success

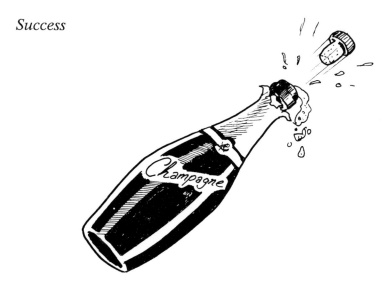

- *Patient*: interest, involvement and participation based on careful promotion of the exercise and personal stimulation and encouragement

- *Staff*: belief and interest in the programme and whole-hearted willingness to be involved

- *Practice team* to accept given roles, to collaborate in details and to accept a period of preparation and training pilot exercises

- *Policies and protocols* to be agreed and adhered to but periodically reviewed

- *Facilities and resources* to be defined and made available

- *Cross-referrals* within the practice and outsiders to be quick and effective

Non-success

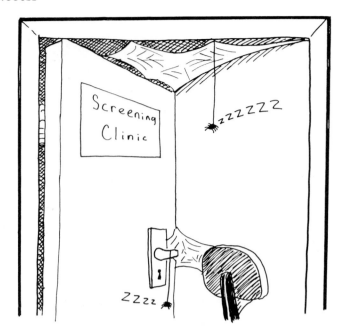

- *Patients* reluctant to attend and at inconvenient times; failure of practice team to promote and encourage the exercise

- *Staff:* less than total acceptance and commitment and disbelief in the whole concept of screening

- *Team:* conflicts of roles

- *Organisation:* inadequate training, no pilot trials and lack of directive leadership

- *All:* boredom and complacency.

Chapter 7

WHITE PAPER AND GP CONTRACT: IMPLICATIONS

Running through the White Paper of 1989 are many issues and items directly related to the principles and policies of 'screening'.

Thus, there is repeated stress on 'health promotion and disease prevention' including early diagnosis, screening, audit, value for money and patient needs and participation.

Since all these activities are to be related to income, it behoves practices to consider, prepare and organise themselves to meet these new challenges and new forms of remuneration.

Most of the screening activities have been noted, but it is useful to set them down again with a few comments.

Ante-natal clinics

This is the first of the screening clinics in which general practice has become involved.

General practice is very well placed to carry out this work in close collaboration with the local obstetric unit. Women come to have their pregnancy confirmed, they are then given an appointment for the practice ante-natal clinic, as well as being referred to the obstetric unit; at the practice clinic the expectant mother also meets the attached community midwife and health visitor, and over the succeeding months will come to know well the practice team.

Good general practice ante-natal care is the best preparation for good child care and surveillance.

CHILD CARE

Transition from ante-natal care to regular practice child care and surveillance should be smooth and easy, for it will be the same doctor and health visitor who will continue to care for the child. It should be up to the health visitor to ensure regular attendance.

A doctor undertaking child surveillance will need to be included on the child health surveillance list and his/her name approved by the FPC; he/she having satisfied the committee that he/she has the required experience and training to undertake this procedure.

NEW ENTRANTS

All new entrants of the practice will need to be invited to attend the practice within 28 days of their acceptance and the following details completed:

1. full medical history
2. lifestyle
3. details of current state of health
4. undertake physical examination including:
   - height   - BP
   - weight   - urinalysis

ELDERLY

All patients over the age of 75 years are to be invited to attend the practice or offered a home visit for an assessment that shall include the following:

1. sensory testing
2. mobility
3. mental condition
4. physical condition
5. continence
6. social involvement
7. review of medication

HEALTH PROMOTION CLINICS

General practitioners are required as part of their general medical services to offer advice to patients about health education which will need to cover the full range of lifestyle activities.

It is mandatory that all practices from 1st April, 1990 produce a practice leaflet giving comprehensive details of the doctors working in the practice including:

– the doctor's year of registration
– the doctor's full medical qualifications

Information will be required about the location of the practice and the extent of the practice boundaries.

The leaflet will need to contain details of the support staff in the practice and full spectrum of clinics which the practice provides for its patients, indicating both the mechanics of the appointment system, repeat prescriptions and out-of-hours consultations.

ANNUAL REPORTS

General practitioners will be required to produce an annual report for the FPC, the first of which must reach the committee by 30th June, 1991 in respect of the year 1st April, 1990–31st March, 1991.

The report will need to include details of staff employed, including their individual details and the qualifications and training of each employee. The report will need to include all the specialities available within the practice and any variations that are planned for the following 12 months.

Details of hospital referrals for both in-patients and out-patients will need to be identified in specific specialities as well as referral rates for X-ray and pathological investigations.

The doctor will be required to identify any commitments undertaken outside the practice and he/she will need to indicate the mechanism in operation to receive patients' comments about the services provided.

The annual report will also need to indicate the arrangements for repeat prescriptions for patients.

POSTGRADUATE EDUCATION

If such new programmes and policies are to be introduced, then education and training of the practice teams will be a high priority.

Chapter 8

FUTURE PROSPECTS

General practice is at a crossroads of time. Historically it has passed rapidly in a lifetime from a corner shop (or part of a doctor's residence) cottage industry, with single-handed doctors working in isolation and competition, through a small business period with group practices and health centres, to the present, where we are on the verge of a big business philosophy which is being hastened by the White Paper and New Contract.

ORGANISATION AND ADMINISTRATION

Much more emphasis in the NHS is being put now on efficiency, effectiveness and economics or, ultimately, 'value for money'.

This will involve a certain loss of free enterprise for general practitioners and Family Practitioner Committees exercising more checks, controls and directives based on more data and information from practices.

To meet such a changing world, general practice will have to become much more business orientated with sharp financial advice and cost-controls.

SHARING

With increasing demands from new roles and tasks requiring more tools, equipment, staff and time, it will be difficult for small units, such as single-handed practices and 2–3 doctor partnerships, to remain profitable and cost-effective.

A radical reconstruction of policies and methods is required. There has to be much closer collaboration and sharing between all those providing health care. No longer should isolated independent practitioners and practices compete for patients; no longer should there be such a cut-off between hospital and general practice; no longer should practices be remote from the life and needs of their local community; and no longer should the people, the patients, be excluded from the policies and organisation of the health care provided for them.

Thus, health care and maintenance, and management of common diseases should be a joint concern of hospital and general practice workers. There should be joint planning and development of protocols for management of asthma, diabetes, high blood pressure, heart attacks, strokes, cancer, terminal care and other conditions. This will have to involve hospital consultants coming out into the community and general practitioners going back into the hospitals. True sharing of care in a planned manner should lead to better and more effective and economic services.

With increasing costs of new technologies, growing specialisation and wider use of non-medical members of the practice teams, there should be much more sharing between local practices. Shared computerisation is an obvious example, but so are sharing of new tools such as nebulisers, auto-analysers and even minor surgery and other skills.

Better sharing of care between general practice and its patients should involve greater responsibilities for patients through information, education and incentives.

PRACTICE PERSONNEL

With the development of general practice and the implementation of the GP contract, 1990, the required programmes of care can best be achieved by developing the role of the practice nurse. The practice nurse (RGN) has professional expertise which is essential to the development of primary care and every effort should be made to establish training programmes for her/him to fulfil her/his role to the fullest extent. It is hoped that the educational programme currently being implemented – Project 2000 – will make provision for the training of future practice nurses.

The expanding practice will also need to consider the employment of other professional colleagues including physiotherapists, chiropodists and counsellors.

NEW TECHNOLOGIES

As well as new philosophies, ideas and attitudes, there are new technologies that have to be introduced into general practice.

– *Information technologies:* It is likely that all practices will be 'computerised' by the end of the 20th century. However, it is essential that this new and wonderful tool be used to its great potential. Computerisation in general practice should be part of the national system, using unique patient numbers and all practices linked and cross-relating to their own

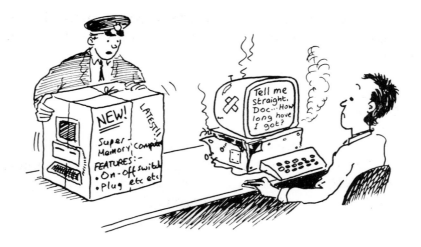

district health data collecting process which must include information from hospital and community services.

– *Industrial technologies:* British general practice has lagged behind in using modern diagnostic and therapeutic technologies because there have been no financial inducements, and because in most districts the services are available through local hospitals. Costings have to be made to see whether it might be cheaper to encourage general practices to have modern equipment which can be shared.

COMMONSENSE PRIORITIES

There has to be planning on priorities. There are finite limits on time and personnel and there have to be priority lists of what is most useful for general practice to undertake in screening to promote health and prevent disease.

The first priority, surely, must be to provide a good personal clinical service that is readily available and accessible. Then in the 'free' time available there will have to be decisions whether all or some, and if so which ones, of these activities should be undertaken:

- child surveillance
- screening of elderly
- new registrant check up
- well-person clinics
- special clinics for cervical cytology, diabetes, high blood pressure, for alcohol and smoking and weight control, pre-natal and genetic advice and others!

Appendix
NATIONAL GROUPS AND ASSOCIATIONS:
Addresses and Telephone Numbers

Age Concern
Bernard Sunley House
60 Pitcairn Road
Mitcham
Surrey
CR4 3LL
Tel. 01 640 5431

Arthritis Care
6 Grosvenor Crescent
London
SW1X 7ER
Tel. 01 235 0902

**Assocation for Spina Bifida
and Hydrocephalus
(ASBAH)**
22 Upper Woburn Place
London
WC1H OEP
Tel. 01 388 1382

Association of Carers
21-23 New Road
Chatham
Kent
ME4 4QJ
Tel. (0634) 013981

Asthma Research Council
300 Upper Street
London
N1 2XX
Tel. 01 226 2260

Alzheimer's Disease
3rd Floor
Bank Buildings
Fulham Broadway
London
SW6 1EP
Tel. 01 381 3177

British Diabetic Association
10 QueenAnne Street
London
W1M OBD
Tel. 01 323 1531

British Dyslexia Assocation
Church Lane
Peppard
Oxon.
RG9 5JN
Tel. 049 17699

British Epilepsy Association
Anstey House
40 Hanover Square
Leeds
LS3 1BE
Tel. 0532 439393

**British Colostomy
Association**
38-39 Eccleston Square
London
SW1V 1PS
Tel. 01 8282 5175

Cruse
Bereavement Care
Cruse House
126 Sheen Road
Richmond
Surrey
TW9 1UR
Tel. 01 940 4818

**Chest, Heart and Stroke
Association**
Tavistock House North
Tavistock Square
London
WC1M 9JE
Tel. 01 387 3012

Disabled Drivers' Assocation
Ashwellthorpe Hall
Ashwellthorpe
Norwich
Norfolk
NR16 1EX
Tel. 050 841 449

Disablement Services Branch
6a Government Buildings
Warbreck Hill Road
Blackpool
FY2 OUZ

Dyslexia Trust
133 Gresham Road
Staines
Middlesex
TW18 2AJ
Tel. 0784 59498

Gamblers Anonymous
17/23 Blantyre Street
Cheyne Walk
London
SW10
Tel. 01 352 3060

Health Education Council
78 New Oxford Street
London
WC1A 1AH
Tel. 01 631 0930

**Hodgkin's Disease
Assocation**
PO Box 275
Haddenham
Aylesbury
Bucks.
HP17 8JJ
Tel. 0602 622382

Leukaemia Society
45 Craigmoor Avenue
Queen's Park
Bournemouth
Dorset
Tel. 0202 374459

**London Voluntary Service
Council**
68 Charlton Street
London
NW1 1JR
Tel. 01 388 0241

Muscular Dystrophy Group
Nattrass House
Macaulay Road
London
SW4
Tel. 01 720 8055

Multiple Sclerosis Society
25 Effin Road
London
SW6 1EE
Tel. 01 736 6267/78

Mobility Information Service
Unit 2a
Atcham Estate
Upton Magna
Shrewsbury
SY4 4UB
Tel. 074 377 489

**National Association for
Mental Health (MIND)**
22 Harley Street
London
W1N 2ED
Tel. 01 637 0741

Mencap
Royal Society for Mentally
Handicapped Children and
Adults
123 Golden Lane
London EC1
Tel. 01 253 9433

**National Assocation of
Disablement Information
and Advice Lines (DIAL UK)**
Victoria Buildings
117 High Street
Clay Cross
Chesterfield
Derbyshire
S45 9DZ
Tel. 0246 250055

**Parkinson's Disease Society
of the UK**
36 Portland Place
London
W1N 3DG
Tel. 01 255 2432

**Royal Association for
Disability and Rehabilitation
(RADAR)**
25 Mortimer Street
London
W1N 8AB
Tel. 01 637 5400

**Royal National Institute for
the Blind**
224 Great Portland Street
London
W1
Tel. 01 388 1266

**Royal National Institute for
the Deaf**
105 Gower Street
London
WC1
Tel. 01 387 8033

Spastics Society
12 Park Crescent
London
W1N 4EQ
Tel. 01 636 5020

Spinal Injuries Association
Newpoint House
76 St. James's Avenue
London
N10 3DF
Tel. 01 444 2121

**Voluntary Council for
Handicapped Children**
National Children's Bureau
8 Wakley Street
London
EC1V 7QE
Tel. 01 278 9441

INDEX

129